REVERSING LIVER FIBROSIS

PREVENTING FURTHER LIVER DAMAGE

Dr. Andrew McPherson

Contents

CHAPTER ONE 4
- PROLOGUE TO REVERSAL OF LIVER FIBROSIS 4
- PATHOBIOLOGY OF HEPATIC FIBROSIS 5
- HEPATIC AGGRAVATION 8
- ROS GENERATION 10

CHAPTER TWO 12
- CYTOKINES 12
- REACTIONS OF THE DIFFERING CELLS OF THE LIVER 13
- REACTIONS DURING FUNDAMENTAL IRRITATION AND INTESTINAL DYSBIOSIS 20
- AUTOPHAGY... 22
- JOB OF MICRORNAS IN FIBROGENESIS 25

CHAPTER THREE 28
- OUTCOMES OF HSC ACTUATION 28
- EVIDENCE OF THE REGRESSION OF FIBROSIS 29
- APOPTOSIS OR INACTIVATION OF HSCS 32

CHAPTER FOUR 36
- CLINICAL EVIDENCE OF REVERSIBILITY ACCORDING TO ETIOLOGY............................ 36

HEPATITIS B INFECTION RELATED LIVER SICKNESS 37

HEPATITIS C INFECTION RELATED LIVER MALADY 42

CHAPTER FIVE 44

ALCOHOLIC LIVER AILMENT 44

NON-ALCOHOLIC GREASY LIVER MALADY ... 45

IMMUNE SYSTEM HEPATITIS 51

CHAPTER SIX 53

ESSENTIAL BILIARY CIRRHOSIS 53

HEMOCHROMATOSIS 56

NEW ANTIFIBROTIC DRUGS AND EXPECTATIONS FOR CLINICAL USE 57

IN A NUTSHELL 62

COULD LIVER FIBROSIS TURNED AROUND? . 64

HOW GENUINE IS FIBROSIS OF THE LIVER? . 64

WHAT ARE THE 4 PHASES OF LIVER AILMENT? 65

THE END 67

CHAPTER ONE

PROLOGUE TO REVERSAL OF LIVER FIBROSIS

Numerous liver sicknesses happen as a reaction to damage over an all-encompassing timeframe before finishing in liver cirrhosis. In spite of the fact that the etiologies of liver illnesses may shift, fibrosis and cirrhosis create through normal flagging pathways. Falls of responses invigorate peaceful hepatic stellate cells (HSCs) into their enacted structures, prompting the collection of collagen and other extracellular lattice (ECM) segments. Supported incitement and amassing of these materials lead to the devastation of liver structures and hepatic innervation, and diminished liver capacity. We have as of late expanded our comprehension of the systems hidden hepatic fibrosis, which might be utilized as potential treatment focuses for the hindrance or inversion of fibrosis. In this audit, we will talk about some new parts of the pathophysiology of fibrosis, the clinical proof of reversibility as indicated by etiology, and future therapeutics for fibrosis.

PATHOBIOLOGY OF HEPATIC FIBROSIS

Enactment of HSCs: a key driving component

Liver fibrogenesis is started by HSC actuation, which is the essential effector cell coordinating the testimony of ECM in the liver structure. HSCs are situated in the perisinusoidal space between the sinusoids and hepatocytes, known as the space of Disse. HSCs actuate the insusceptible reaction through the discharge of cytokines and chemokines and through associations with invulnerable cells. Initiation of HSCs can be incited by a scope of constant liver provocative variables, receptive oxygen species (ROS), and cytokines. Actuated HSCs are changed into myofibroblasts, which have profibrogenic properties; they emit changing development factor β (TGF-β), α-smooth muscle actin, and type I collagen.

Procedure of hepatic stellate cell (HSC) separation during movement and relapse of fibrosis. In the fundamental pathway of liver fibrosis, HSCs experience separation from peaceful cells to myofibroblasts. A neighboring situation that is portrayed by various safe cells, cytokines, and little atoms organizes this procedure. TGF-β, changing development factor β; CCL2, C-C theme chemokine ligand type 2; IL, interleukin; TNF-α, tumor rot factor α; PDGF, platelet-inferred development factor; MMP, network metalloproteinase; CB1, cannabinoid receptor 1; PPAR-γ, peroxisome proliferator-enacted receptor γ; NK, normal executioner.

HEPATIC AGGRAVATION

Constant aggravation is the primary driver of hepatic fibrogenesis and it was seen as present in most of ceaseless liver sicknesses, for example, viral hepatitis, harmful liver damage, alcoholic hepatitis, non-alcoholic steatohepatitis (NASH), and immune system liver maladies. Hepatic aggravation brings about actuation of HSCs through a few components and pathways regardless of its etiology. Introductory paracrine incitement, including presentation to apoptotic assemblages of harmed hepatocytes can, thus, initiate peaceful HSCs and change them into myofibroblasts. Lipid peroxides from Kupffer cells drive early initiation and changes in the encompassing ECM.

Lipopolysaccharide (LPS) enacts Toll-like receptor 4 motioning in Kupffer cells prompting the actuation of atomic factor κ-light-chain-enhancer of initiated B cells (NF-κB)- interferon administrative factor 3 pathway and the ensuing transcriptional actuation of proinflammatory cytokines, for example, tumor rot factor α (TNF-α) and interferon γ (IFN-γ). This pathway prompts endothelial cell brokenness, hindered trade of solutes among neighboring cells, modified hepatocyte work, and ensuing non-parenchymal cell harm. In an exploratory investigation, HSCs demonstrated a progressively enacted phenotype, more noteworthy expansion rates, and expanded collagen blend when they were co-refined with Kupffer cells or hepatocytes, when contrasted with when they were refined alone.

ROS GENERATION

ROS discharged by Kupffer cells and hepatocytes can expand oxidative worry in hepatocytes, advance their apoptosis, and further animate the initiation of HSCs. ROS are created primarily by means of the mitochondrial electron transport chain or by means of enactment of cytochrome P450, nicotinamide adenine dinucleotide phosphate (NADPH) oxidase, xanthine oxidase, or by means of mitochondrial harm. The creation of ROS is impacted by the movement of NADPH oxidase in HSCs, macrophages, and hepatocytes and by the generation of nitric oxide in Kupffer cells. Clinically in drunkards, there is a solid acceptance of cytochrome P450 2E1 prompting expanded ROS and pericentral (zone 3) harm. NADPH oxidase intervenes liver damage and fibrosis through the age of oxidative pressure.

CHAPTER TWO

CYTOKINES

Cytokines, including TGF-β, platelet-inferred development factor (PDGF), and endothelial development factor prompt the change of quiet HSCs into myofibroblasts. Angiotensin II, which is emitted by HSCs, improves HSC multiplication and, thusly, adds to the generation of ECM. The cannabinoid receptor cannabinoid receptor 1 (CB1) is upregulated in myofibroblasts or initiated HSCs, and builds hepatic fibrosis. Interestingly, the CB2 receptor on these cells shows an antifibrotic impact. Furthermore, adipokines likewise add to the hepatic signs of weight and fibrogenesis. Leptin, which is a coursing adipogenic hormone, advances stellate cell fibrogenesis, improves tissue inhibitor of metalloproteinase 1 (TIMP-1) articulation, applies its activity through Janus kinase (JAK)-signal transduction, and smothers peroxisome proliferator-initiated receptor γ (PPAR-γ).

Invulnerable reactions: variable jobs in hepatic fibrosis

Invulnerable associations assume a significant job in driving fibrogenesis, as tireless irritation as a rule goes before fibrosis.

REACTIONS OF THE DIFFERING CELLS OF THE LIVER

Enacted HSCs discharge incendiary cytokines,

communicate legitimately with insusceptible cells by communicating distinctive grip particles, and adjust the versatile safe framework by working as antigen showing cells. In this way, a positive criticism circle exists in which fiery and fibrogenic cells animate each other to intensify fibrosis. Other cell types that control the movement and goals of fibrosis incorporate liver sinusoidal endothelial cells (LSECs), Kupffer cells, hepatocytes, regular executioner (NK) cells, T cells, monocytes, cholangiocytes, ductular cells, entrance fibroblasts, and different other fiery cells.

Hepatic revascularization with LSEC actuation and expansion is exceptionally connected with perisinusoidal fibrosis. During perisinusoidal fibrosis, enacted LSECs add to ECM generation including amalgamation of storm cellar film segments, fibronectin, and interstitial collagen type 1. They additionally produce cytokines that initiate HSCs and emit factors that add to intrahepatic vasoconstriction, which adds to entry hypertension in cirrhosis.

Kupffer cell actuation prompts expanded NF-κB movement and ensuing discharge of proinflammatory cytokines and chemokines including TNF-α and monocyte chemoattractant protein 1 (MCP-1). Thusly, HSCs react to this incitement by emitting macrophage state animating element, MCP-1, interleukin 6 (IL-6), C-C theme chemokine ligand type 21 (CCL21), and C-C theme chemokine receptor type 5 (CCR5) prompting an intensified intense stage reaction with further initiation of macrophages. TNF-α likewise initiates neutrophil penetration and animates mitochondrial oxidant creation in hepatocytes, which experience apoptosis. Harm to hepatocytes, which happens transcendently in liver maladies portrayed by upgraded oxidative and endoplasmic reticulum stress, lysosomal enactment, and mitochondrial harm, are a solid trigger for fibrogenesis. Phagocytosis of harmed hepatocytes by myofibroblasts triggers their fibrogenic initiation through NADPH oxidase 2 and the JAK/signal transducer and activator of translation (STAT) and phosphoinositide 3-kinase/Akt pathways.

NK cells apply their antifibrotic movement by restraining and murdering initiated HSCs. In liver damage, NK cells instigate apoptosis of HSCs through the generation of IFN-γ, despite the fact that this pathway can't be actuated in cutting edge phases of liver fibrosis. HSCs interface legitimately with different safe cells by communicating bond particles including intercellular attachment atom 1 and vascular cell grip particle 1. The declaration of both of these attachment atoms is expanded in HSCs during damage, which is interceded by TNF-α, and tops with maximal cell penetration. Along these lines, bond atom enlistment on HSCs encourages the enrollment of fiery cells to the harmed liver.

CD4+ T cells with a Th2 polarization advance fibrogenesis in the liver, lungs, and kidneys. Th2 cells, specifically, produce IL-4 and IL-13, which invigorate the separation of possibly fibrogenic myeloid cells and initiated macrophages. In test considers, rodents with Th2-prevailing T cell penetration show quick fibrosis movement, while CD4+ Th1 cells have an antifibrotic impact.

Monocytes assume a key job in aggravation and fibrosis. They are likewise forerunners of fibrocytes, macrophages, and dendritic cells (DCs), and offer qualities with myeloid silencer cells. At the interface of intrinsic and versatile resistance, monocytes help versatile invulnerable reactions, and proinflammatory monocytes (CD14+ and CD16+ in people) advance fibrogenesis. Communication among chemokines and their receptors is significant in the enrollment, initiation, and capacity of monocytes; it could be an appealing objective for fibrosis tweak. CCL2 and its receptor CCR2 are key to monocyte enrollment to the liver during hepatic aggravation and fibrosis. Despite the fact that their hindrance enhances fibrosis movement in rat models, they additionally defer fibrosis inversion. Monocytes are the antecedents of flowing fibrocytes, which are cells that separate into collagen-creating fibroblasts, and are identified with bone marrow (BM) mesenchymal undifferentiated cells (MSCs). Furthermore, monocytes are the wellspring of fibrolytic CD133+ cells that gather in the liver to initiate fibrosis inversion after BM transplantation. Chemokines and their receptors are significant in monocyte enrollment and initiation, speaking to appealing focuses for fibrosis adjustment.

REACTIONS DURING FUNDAMENTAL IRRITATION AND INTESTINAL DYSBIOSIS

During fundamental irritation, the insusceptible reaction is started when microorganisms are presented through gateway stream from the intestinal lumen. Pathogen-related sub-atomic examples (PAMPs) from enteric bacterial life forms and harm related sub-atomic examples (DAMPs) beginning from the host tissue upon damage invigorate intrinsic safe cells. Safe acknowledgment of microbes and PAMPs including LPS, lipopeptides, glycopolymers, flagellin, and bacterial DNA happens both locally in the gut-related lymph hub tissue (GALT) and in mesenteric lymph hubs (MLN) just as fundamentally. Moreover, insusceptible cells previously enacted in the GALT and MLN may enter the fringe blood and spread the incendiary reaction foundationally. DAMPs and sterile particulates, likewise discharged from necrotic hepatocytes, may likewise add to inspire a provocative reaction and fibrosis.

Intracellular reaction during hepatic fibrogenesis

AUTOPHAGY

Autophagy takes an interest in hepatic fibrosis by initiating HSCs and may likewise partake by impacting other fibrogenic cells. Calm HSCs are loaded up with cytoplasmic lipid beads (LDs) that contain retinyl esters. Alongside the change from LD-rich cells to myofibroblast-like cells, autophagy transition is upregulated. Autophagy may supply vitality for initiation of HSCs by conveying triglycerides and different segments in LDs from autophagosomes to lysosomes for corruption.

Actuation of TGF-β and the Smad pathway

In the liver, the job of TGF-β is significant because of its different consequences for hepatocellular multiplication and liver recovery, acceptance of parenchymal cell apoptosis, insusceptible observation, and hepatic fibrogenesis. Also, TGF-β discharged by myofibroblasts can instigate hepatocellular apoptosis after actuation. During fibrogenesis, tissue and blood levels of dynamic TGF-β are raised and overexpression of TGF-β1 can instigate fibrosis. These impacts, alongside the capacity of TGF-β to upregulate ECM articulation and the nearness of useful TGF-β receptors on the outside of HSCs with persevering autocrine incitement of enacted HSCs and myofibroblasts by TGF-β, are key systems of liver fibrogenesis. In view of the distinguishing proof of downstream occasions of TGF-β flagging transduction in the course of recent years, TGF-β1 has been appeared to initiate Smad2 and Smad3, which are adversely managed by Smad7, an inhibitor of TGF-β motioning, through the ubiquitin-proteasome corruption system. With regards to liver fibrosis, Smad3 is profibrogenic, as Smad3 knockout mice are ensured against dimethylnitrosamine-prompted hepatic fibrosis. In spite of the fact that Smad7 exhaustion advances hepatic fibrosis, Smad7 is defensive since its overexpression secures against HSC enactment and hepatic fibrosis in vitro and in vivo examinations.

JOB OF MICRORNAS IN FIBROGENESIS

MicroRNAs (miRNA) speak to a group of little non-coding RNAs that control the interpretation and translation of numerous qualities. Dysregulation of miRNA influences a wide scope of cell procedures, for example, cell multiplication and separation engaged with organ renovating forms. The significance of miR-29 in hepatic collagen homeostasis is underlined by in vivo information showing that test serious fibrosis is related with a conspicuous miR-

29 reduction. The loss of miR-29 is because of the reaction of HSCs to presentation to the profibrogenic go betweens TGF-β and PDGF. A few putative restricting locales for the Smad proteins and the Ap1 complex are situated in the miR-29 advertiser, which are proposed to intercede the lessening in miR-29 in fibrosis. Different miRNAs are profoundly expanded after profibrogenic incitement, for example, miR-21. miR-21 is transcriptionally upregulated in light of Smad3 instead of Smad2 enactment after TGF-β incitement. What's more, TGF-β advances miR-21 articulation by development of a microchip complex containing Smad proteins. Raised miR-21 may then go about as a profibrogenic miRNA by curbing

the TGF-β inhibitory Smad7 protein.

CHAPTER THREE

OUTCOMES OF HSC ACTUATION

The ECM is a significant segment of the liver structure and experiences exceptionally unique changes during amalgamation and corruption. Dangerous neurotic conditions emerge when ECM redesigning gets exorbitant or uncontrolled. HSCs, neutrophils, and macrophages are associated with hepatic ECM corruption. Lattice metalloproteinases (MMPs) are the principle compounds liable for ECM debasement and TIMPs can restrain MMPs. Subsequently, guideline of the MMP-TIMP equalization is basic for effective ECM redesigning. Initiated HSCs not just incorporate and discharge

ECM proteins, for example, type I and type III collagen yet in addition produce MMP1 and MMP13. Additionally, enacted HSCs up-direct the articulation and union of TIMP1 and TIMP2. TIMP1 not just avoids the corruption of the quickly expanding ECM by blocking MMPs yet additionally hinders apoptosis of enacted HSCs. The net outcome is the testimony of full grown collagen filaments inside the space of Disse, bringing about scarring.

EVIDENCE OF THE REGRESSION OF FIBROSIS

Increment in fibrolytic movement

The enlistment and ensuing unconstrained goals of fibrosis has been seen in a few creature models, and comprise information that are priceless in deciding the fundamental natural components of fibrosis. Despite ECM debasement, fibrotic ECM keeps on aggregating in interminable liver damage as a result of restraint of MMP movement by myofibroblast-inferred TIMP-1. A few studies researching the goals of liver fibrosis in rodents indicated that degrees of TIMP-1 diminished after the suspension of damage. As the degree of TIMP-1 diminished, hepatic collagenase action expanded and ECM debasement happened. Ensuing unthinking thinks about that modified TIMP to adjust MMP levels in situ have affirmed the amazing impact of this proportion on the advancement and goals of fibrosis in the liver. As far as rebuilding of macrophages, macrophages have likewise been demonstrated to be urgent in the goals of fibrosis, which underlines their job as controllers of viable injury mending and organ homeostasis. Situated in fibrotic tissue of the liver, macrophages are unmistakably set to intervene ECM corruption and are a rich wellspring of fibrolytic MMPs, including MMP12/13. Macrophages additionally express TNF-related apoptosis-initiating ligand that advances myofibroblast apoptosis. Moreover, phagocytosis of apoptotic cells by macrophages initiates MMP articulation and enlarges ECM debasement in rat models of settling hepatocellular fibrosis. Adjustment of DCs has likewise been researched with regards to the goals of liver fibrosis utilizing Cd11c-diphtheria poison receptor (DTR) transgenic mice to drain hepatic DCs during the recuperation stage, following CCl4-intervened damage, just as the utilization of supportive exchange conventions. DCs were appeared to intercede ECM debasement, most likely through upgraded MMP9 articulation.

APOPTOSIS OR INACTIVATION OF HSCS

Actuation of HSCs in light of incessant liver damage is a key advance in the pathogenesis of liver fibrosis. As of late, clinical and test studies have exhibited that fibrosis goals may endless supply of the liver affront. Exploratory models of fibrosis recuperation have reliably detailed that disposal of actuated HSCs by apoptosis or inactivation of fibrolytic pathways prompted the relapse of fibrosis. This recommends freedom of actuated HSCs is a key advance in the beginning of fibrosis relapse. Myofibroblasts produce sinewy scars in hepatic fibrosis. In the CCl4 model of liver fibrosis, calm HSCs are initiated and changed into myofibroblasts. At the point when the basic etiological operator is evacuated, clinical and test fibrosis experience a surprising relapse, with complete vanishing of these myofibroblasts. In any case, it was indicated that a subset of the myofibroblasts got away apoptosis during relapse of liver fibrosis, down-directed fibrogenic qualities, and gained a phenotype like, however particular from, quiet HSCs; they had the option to all the more quickly reactivate into myofibroblasts because of fibrogenic improvements and emphatically add to liver fibrosis. Inactivation of HSCs was related with up-guideline of antiapoptotic qualities, for example, Hspa1a/b, which take part in the endurance of HSCs in culture and in vivo.

To sum things up, liver fibrosis as a rule has potential for relapse. Early liver fibrosis, which needs ECM crosslinking and checked angiogenesis, can even invert into practically ordinary design if the fundamental cause is effectively treated. This is viewed as the best type of antifibrotic treatment and encourages the consequent endogenous guideline of wound mending.

CHAPTER FOUR

CLINICAL EVIDENCE OF REVERSIBILITY ACCORDING TO ETIOLOGY

Relapse of fibrosis is currently a reality in clinical settings. The sequential appraisal of biopsy tests from patients with interminable liver sickness of various etiologies, who were effectively treated, shows that liver fibrosis is a dynamic and bidirectional procedure that has a characteristic limit with respect to recuperation and renovating. Next, we will depict the proof and research results of liver fibrosis recuperation in clinical practice settings as indicated by various etiologies.

HEPATITIS B INFECTION RELATED LIVER SICKNESS

Constant hepatitis B (CHB) is a huge overall issue as CHB patients create cirrhosis and hepatocellular carcinoma. Standard medicines incorporate pegylated IFN-α and nucleostide analogs. A few studies have exhibited that hepatitis B infection (HBV) DNA concealment is related with biochemical and histological reactions. There is presently proof that these surrogate markers relate with improved long haul clinical result. IFN has been utilized in the treatment of CHB since the 1980s. Peginterferon treatment has been appeared to diminish fibrosis movement in hepatitis B encompass antigen (HBeAg)- positive patients, with a more noteworthy reaction found in the individuals who continue HBeAg seroconversion, just as in HBeAg negative patients with a supported virologic/biochemical reaction. In one exploratory examination, IFN-α treatment showed antifibrotic movement by repressing the generation of TGF-β, diminishing HSC actuation, and invigorating HSC apoptosis in vitro. Another study watched the antifibrotic impact that IFN-γ applied in liver cells through STAT-1 phosphorylation and hindered TGF-β flagging. Long haul treatment with nucleoside analogs has additionally been appeared to improve liver fibrosis and malady movement. In a 3-year investigation of lamivudine for hepatitis B treatment, follow-up liver biopsies demonstrated inversion of cirrhosis in eight of 11 patients (73%). Entecavir, which is an increasingly intense inhibitor of viral replication in CHB, improves liver fibrosis. In an ongoing report, 96% of patients had histological improvement after long haul treatment with entecavir. Ten of the 57 patients had propelled fibrosis or cirrhosis (Ishak score 4 to 6) at pattern. Each of the 10 patients accomplished in any event a 1-point decrease in the Ishak fibrosis score after long haul entecavir treatment. In a later 5-year study with tenofovir treatment for constant HBV contamination that included patients with liver cirrhosis toward the beginning of the examination, 74% showed broad histological improvement, to such an extent that they were never again viewed as cirrhotic.

As of late, rather than liver biopsy, transient elastography (TE) has been applied for the clinical evaluation of liver fibrosis. An enormous imminent partner investigation of 426 people announced a noteworthy decrease in TE esteems in CHB patients following 3 years of antiviral treatment. Be that as it may, the critical decrease in TE esteems at development, contrasted with those at pattern, was restricted in patients who had at first raised alanine transaminase (ALT) levels. To bar the perplexing impact of high ALT, another examination explored changes in TE esteems during antiviral treatment in 41 patients with CHB showing low ALT levels (≤ 2 × the maximum furthest reaches of ordinary).

Following 1 to 2 years of antiviral treatment, TE esteems essentially diminished contrasted and gauge, though ALT levels stayed unaltered. Non-intrusive serum fibrosis markers were likewise used for the appraisal of changes in liver fibrosis. It was accounted for that fibrosis dependent on the four components (FIB-4) and the aspartate aminotransferase-to-platelet proportion file (APRI) were altogether improved in 370 HBV-related cirrhosis patients who got 2 years of entecavir treatment. These outcomes propose that potential fibrosis relapse could be conceivable with long haul antiviral treatment and that clinical checking utilizing non-intrusive techniques is helpful.

HEPATITIS C INFECTION RELATED LIVER MALADY

Patients with remunerated cirrhosis and ceaseless hepatitis C (CHC) advantage from IFN-based antiviral treatment. Viral annihilation can be accomplished in up to 40% of patients with genotype 1, and in 70% of patients with genotypes 2 or 3, diminishing the danger of creating cirrhosis, hepatic decompensation, and hepatocellular carcinoma. In a 5-year line up investigation of CHC patients with organize 2 or more prominent fibrosis at benchmark, 82% of patients who had accomplished supported virologic reaction (SVR) after IFN treatment had diminished fibrosis scores. Another concentrate showed a decrease in clinical occasions after SVR. Notwithstanding IFN, amazing viability has been accounted for with a few new straightforwardly acting antiviral operators (DAA) for HCV. Albeit little information were accounted for on follow-up liver biopsy, an ongoing report indicated the plausibility of inversion of liver fibrosis and cirrhosis by circuitous estimation. TE esteems just as FIB-4 and APRI scores were assessed before treatment and inside year and a half after DAA treatment; patients who had accomplished SVR after DAA treatment indicated critical relapse of TE esteems and improvement of FIB-4 and APRI scores. Liver fibrosis and cirrhosis are relied upon to improve in these patients with goals of HCV disease.

CHAPTER FIVE

ALCOHOLIC LIVER AILMENT

Clinical proof for relapse of fibrosis in alcoholic liver malady is constrained. Results from randomized controlled preliminaries (RCTs) surveying the impacts of pharmacological specialists on alcoholic fibrosis and cirrhosis have been baffling. A Cochrane Intervention Review evaluating the impact of colchicine for alcoholic and non-alcoholic liver fibrosis and cirrhosis from 15 RCTs revealed the nonappearance of measurably noteworthy upgrades in any critical clinical result, including liver histology. Be that as it may, there is a slight impact of forbearance of liquor on clinical result. In one investigation, 100 patients with alcoholic cirrhosis were pursued for a long time after their benchmark histological appraisal. Forbearance at multi month post-biopsy was related with a critical improvement in long haul endurance. This article exhibited that there were advantages of forbearance after longer development, with factually noteworthy contrasts in 5-year endurance rates between the individuals who avoided and persevering fermented consumers (75% and half, separately; p < 0.002).

NON-ALCOHOLIC GREASY LIVER MALADY

There are right now no affirmed medicines for non-alcoholic greasy liver ailment (NAFLD) and treatments are in view of focusing on hazard factors. Despite the fact that there have been a few investigations characterizing the advantages of different pharmacological specialists for NAFLD, these examinations have been constrained by little examination populaces and present moment follow-up periods. Weight decrease through way of life alteration is the principal treatment methodology in NAFLD patients. Weight decrease is frequently connected with valuable consequences for numerous parts of metabolic disorder. Histological enhancements have likewise been watched, especially as for steatosis, yet proof of fibrosis relapse is disputable. A RCT evaluating the impact of weight decrease through way of life adjustment in 31 NASH patients over a 48-week time frame exhibited huge upgrades in the NASH histological action score following a normal weight reduction of 9.3%, however neglected to show a huge change in fibrosis.

Supplementation with the common type of nutrient E (800 IU/day) has helpful impacts in patients with NASH, yet advantages of pioglitazone are less clear as indicated by the most recent discoveries from the Pioglitazone versus Nutrient E versus Fake treatment for the Treatment of Nondiabetic Patients with Nonalcoholic Steatohepatitis (PIVENS) preliminary. In this examination, 247 grown-ups with biopsy-affirmed NASH without diabetes mellitus were haphazardly doled out to one of the three after treatment gatherings: (1) 30 mg for each day of pioglitazone notwithstanding fake treatment; (2) 800 IU of nutrient E every day notwithstanding fake treatment; and (3) two fake treatment tablets day by day. The essential result was a composite of progress in hepatocellular swelling, no declining of fibrosis, and improved movement scores for NASH. Twice the same number of patients treated with nutrient E accomplished the essential result contrasted with the individuals who got fake treatment (43% versus 19%). Albeit a greater number of patients in the pioglitazone bunch than the fake treatment gathering satisfied the essential result (34% versus 19%), the thing that matters was not measurably critical.

An ongoing fake treatment controlled randomized preliminary exhibited that obeticholic corrosive, an engineered farnesoid X receptor agonist, was successful in patients with NASH. Patients were treated for 72 weeks and the essential endpoint was improvement in histology, as estimated by a two-point decrease in a composite movement histological score without exacerbating of fibrosis. The helpful period of the preliminary was halted early incompletely in light of the fact that a preplanned between time examination uncovered that more patients on obeticholic corrosive (45%, 50 of 110) than on fake treatment (21%, 23 of 109) arrived at the essential endpoint (relative hazard, 1.9; 95% certainty interim, 1.3 to 2.8). Thirty-six of 102 obeticholic corrosive treated patients (35%) exhibited fibrosis relapse by one phase or more contrasted with 19 of 98 fake treatment treated patients (19%). In spite of the fact that the investigation was halted after the between time examination, the fundamental aftereffect of this investigation shows a reasonable improvement in every single histological component of NASH, including steatosis, irritation, and liver-cell damage, together with a decrease in aminotransferases, biochemical markers of hepatic harm.

IMMUNE SYSTEM HEPATITIS

Roughly 40% of patients with immune system hepatitis create cirrhosis under current treatments. Despite the fact that the course is variable relying upon the time of perception, the yearly event of cirrhosis is evaluated at 3% every year. A few studies have not just shown the antifibrotic impacts of immunosuppressive treatment in immune system hepatitis yet have additionally fortified the relationship between the files of hepatic aggravation and the movement of liver fibrosis. Fibrosis scores utilizing the Ishak framework improved in 46 of 87 treated patients (53%) with immune system hepatitis during 63 months, and the histological movement file diminished simultaneously. They recommended that improvement of hepatic fibrosis is conceivable in most of treated patients with immune system hepatitis and that inability to smother liver aggravation intensifies fibrosis.

CHAPTER SIX

ESSENTIAL BILIARY CIRRHOSIS

The main clinically endorsed therapeutic treatment for essential biliary cirrhosis (PBC) is ursodeoxycholic corrosive (UDCA). Be that as it may, there are discussions with respect to the elucidation of current proof. In a few investigations with hybrid from fake treatment or no UDCA treatment, the hybrid patients' conditions decayed regardless of utilizing UDCA. A Cochrane Review assessing 16 RCTs utilizing UDCA versus fake treatment uncovered that practically 50% of these preliminaries had a high danger of predisposition and inferred that UDCA didn't fundamentally improve liver histology and had no obvious impact on improving mortality. In any case, UDCA may have benefits in beginning time and asymptomatic PBC. In the asymptomatic PBC partner depicted by Prince etal. 45% of the patients taking UDCA didn't create liver-related side effects during a middle follow-up of 7.4 years.

The job of immunosuppressive specialists in PBC stays questionable. A couple of studies assessing methotrexate have introduced clashing outcomes and a few studies recommend that methotrexate may decline mortality.

Obeticholic corrosive, a subsidiary of chenodeoxycholic corrosive, has, not at all like UDCA, solid enacting impacts on the atomic receptor farnesoid X receptor in stage II results. In an ongoing clinical preliminary with obeticholic corrosive as treatment for PBC, great impacts were likewise seen in PBC patients with an insufficient reaction to UDCA. Basic phosphatase, γ glutamyl transpeptidase, and alanine aminotransferase levels were fundamentally improved in patients getting obeticholic corrosive contrasted and those in the fake treatment gathering. In this investigation, the treatment time frame was just 3 months and liver biopsies were not acquired to distinguish histologic changes. Subjects were permitted to partake in an open-mark augmentation preliminary, which showed continued reductions in liver chemical levels more than a year. Future preliminaries to decide the advantageous impacts of obeticholic corrosive on hepatic fibrosis in patients with essential cirrhosis are justified.

HEMOCHROMATOSIS

Not many investigations have distinguished a relapse of fibrosis and inversion of cirrhosis utilizing liver biopsy following phlebotomy in patients with innate hemochromatosis. The latest investigation tending to reversibility of liver fibrosis or cirrhosis evaluated histological result following phlebotomy in 36 instances of C282Y homozygotes with reported F3 or F4 fibrosis on list biopsy. The 36 patients were selected from C282Y homozygotes with either serious fibrosis or cirrhosis (F3 or F4 fibrosis, organized by the METAVIR evaluating framework). When characterizing relapse of fibrosis as an abatement of at any rate 2 METAVIR units, fibrosis relapsed in nine of 13 patients (69%) with organize F3 and in eight of 23 patients (35%) with arrange F4 fibrosis.

NEW ANTIFIBROTIC DRUGS AND EXPECTATIONS FOR CLINICAL USE

As of late, there has been an unfaltering expansion to the quantity of atoms and pathways that are focuses for antifibrotic treatment; TGF-β1 remains the most significant of such particles. Notwithstanding, foundational restraint of TGF-β1 brings about expanded irritation. This has prodded the focusing of explicit strides of TGF-β1 initiation in a confined way. Hindrance of integrin αvβ6, with decrease of TGF-β1 enactment, vows to be an exceptionally viable and limited antifibrotic approach. Connective tissue development factor (CTGF) intensifies TGF-β1 flagging, and a monoclonal neutralizer focusing on CTGF has indicated guarantee in creature models of organ fibrosis. Lessening the initiated phenotype of myofibroblasts is an appealing methodology because of their key job in ECM affidavit. Restraint of the CB1 switches myofibroblast initiation and weakens exploratory liver fibrosis. This has passed the confirmation of guideline state, and fringe acting CB1 foes that may bypass unfriendly symptoms on the focal sensory system, for example, misery, are being created. In fibrotic NASH, movement is personally connected with insulin obstruction/type 2 diabetes just as lipotoxic hepatocyte demise and intestinal dysbiosis, giving reasonable focuses to both calming and antifibrotic treatment. Restorative methodologies incorporate lessening oxidative pressure, improving insulin flagging, enacting the farnesoid X receptor (e.g., with obeticholic corrosive), fibrosis-focused on inhibitors of hedgehog flagging, joined PPAR-α/δ agonists, or control of modified gut microbiota utilizing probiotics or microbiota move. Albeit oxidative pressure is a significant cofactor in fibrosis, the utilization of cancer prevention agents has demonstrated baffling. Initiation of NADPH oxidases (NOX1, NOX 2, and NOX4) actuates HSC enactment. NOX4 can trigger apoptosis in hepatocytes. NOX inhibitors have been read for the aversion of liver fibrosis.

Also, a few applicant particles have been tried in steatohepatitis patients that have a solid preclinical method of reasoning. These incorporate the double PPAR-α/δ (GFT505), CCR1 and CCR5 enemies, antifibrotic specialists (simtuzumab), Takeda G-protein coupled receptor 5

(TGR5) agonists or receptor agonists, and the unsaturated fat bile corrosive conjugate aramchol. The majority of these specialists are as of now in cutting edge stage 2b and stage 3 clinical preliminaries. The medication pipeline is gradually working to address the clinical needs of this quiet yet harming liver illness. As of late, MSC treatment has been proposed as a viable exchange approach for the treatment of hepatic fibrosis. MSCs can possibly separate into hepatocytes and their remedial worth lies in their insusceptible modulatory properties and discharge of trophic elements, for example, development elements and cytokines.

IN A NUTSHELL

Hepatic fibrogenesis is an unpredictable and directed procedure that speaks to the harmony between grid generation and corruption. HSCs are significant factors in the fibrogenic procedure and are a promising objective for antifibrotic treatments. Despite the fact that the resistant framework and HSCs equally manage each other to engender fibrogenesis, an antifibrotic pathway including NK and DCs likewise invigorates HSC apoptosis. In spite of the advances in understanding the components basic hepatic fibrosis, there is a huge slack in applying these to clinical medicines. By and by, progress in the following decade is relied upon to uncover ways to deal with invert fibrosis through further translational research.

Clinically, the most persuading proof for the relapse of liver fibrosis is gotten from enormous scale investigations of antiviral treatments for the treatment of CHC and hepatitis B. Long haul follow-up studies show that relapse of liver fibrosis is related with improved clinical results by reinforcing apparent histological relapse. In spite of the fact that fibrosis relapse stays a dubious subject, we accept that relapse of fibrosis could in the long run be accomplished by explaining the different flagging pathways associated with HSC initiation just as through the utilization of potential new antifibrotic methodologies.

COULD LIVER FIBROSIS TURNED AROUND?

Fibrosis happens when the liver is more than once or consistently harmed or inflammed1. It is a condition that can be turned around whenever seen in the beginning times and steps are taken to counteract further harm. Recognizing and managing the reason can generally accomplish inversion of early fibrosis.

HOW GENUINE IS FIBROSIS OF THE LIVER?

Fibrosis of the Liver. Fibrosis is the development of an anomalous huge measure of scar tissue in the liver. It happens when the liver endeavors to fix and supplant harmed cells. Fibrosis itself causes no indications, yet serious scarring can bring about cirrhosis, which can cause side effects.

WHAT ARE THE 4 PHASES OF LIVER AILMENT?

Phases of liver harm

•   stage 0: no fibrosis.

•   stage 1: mellow fibrosis without dividers of scarring.

•   stage 2: mellow to direct fibrosis with dividers of scarring.

•   stage 3: connecting fibrosis or scarring that has spread to various pieces of the liver however no cirrhosis.

- stage 4: extreme scarring, or cirrhosis.

THE END

Made in United States
North Haven, CT
19 April 2025